Ayurveda For Be

A Guide To The Ancient Practice Of Balance And Natural Health Harmonize Your Body, Soul, And Mind With Simple-To-Follow Ayurvedic Healing Tips

Jimmy D. Forest

Bluesource And Friends

This book is brought to you by Bluesource And Friends, a happy book publishing company.

Our motto is **"Happiness Within Pages"**

We promise to deliver amazing value to readers with our books.

We also appreciate honest book reviews from our readers.

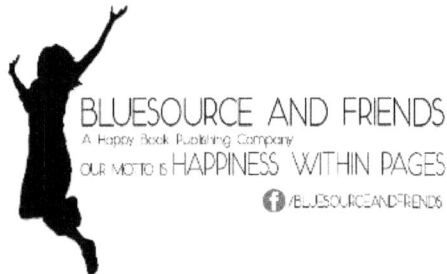

Connect with us on our Facebook page www.facebook.com/bluesourceandfriends and stay tuned to our latest book promotions and free giveaways.

Don't forget to claim your FREE books!

Brain Teasers:

https://tinyurl.com/karenbrainteasers

Harry Potter Trivia:

https://tinyurl.com/wizardworldtrivia

Sherlock Puzzle Book (Volume 2)

https://tinyurl.com/Sherlockpuzzlebook2

Also check out our best seller books

"67 Lateral Thinking Puzzles"

https://tinyurl.com/thinkingandriddles

"Rookstorm Online Saga"

https://tinyurl.com/rookstorm

Table of Contents

Introduction

Congratulations on getting *Ayurveda for Beginners*, and thank you for doing so. This ancient system of medicine is used to maintain our health, and stave off diseases by attuning our lifestyles and diets to fit our unique constitutions. By doing this, we can maintain the balance within, and in turn, maintain our good health. Widely practiced on the Indian subcontinent, Ayurveda has been growing in popularity in the Western world for the past several decades. Although still considered an alternative form of medical treatment, more and more people are beginning to learn the principles of Ayurveda and apply them to their daily lives. Many sources think that the origins of Ayurveda trace all the way back to around 6,000 BCE, when it originated as an oral tradition. In this book, we will dive into the origin and development of Ayurveda and explore how it is commonly practiced in modern times. Every individual is unique in Ayurveda, and we'll learn that the choices we make in terms of our lifestyle and nutrition have the largest impact on our overall health.

The following chapters will discuss the primary principles that make up Ayurveda, and how you can translate them to your daily life. Identifying which dosha you are most influenced by will be the starting point for your new journey. In Ayurveda, everyone has a certain influence of combinations of the five primary elements: Fire, water, earth, air, and space. It's these combinations that form the three energies, or life forces. By determining which of Kapha, Pitta, or Vata dosha you belong to, you can better determine the correct diet and the best courses of action on your path to health and wellness. We'll explore the different ways that you can experiment with Ayurvedic medicine to achieve harmony in body, soul, and mind. This means having an accurate picture of your health, characteristics, and goals. You'll be able to utilize this information on a deeper level if you understand where you are coming from, as well as know how you would like to proceed. There will be tips for healing using Ayurvedic yoga, as well as mantras and chakras. We continue with using Ayurvedic theory in terms of aromatherapy and herbal remedies.

Next, we will determine the different techniques you can use to approach weight loss through Ayurveda. If you've experienced health-related issues, you may want to examine the foods you are eating. Through Ayurveda and the three doshas, we can determine which types of foods are best for every type. Recipes are provided for you to get a jump-start in using Ayurvedic theory for weight-loss and for restoring balance in your life through your diet. You may wish to have an initial assessment with an Ayurvedic practitioner to determine your unique balance of doshas. Once your constitution has been determined, you can come up with individualized treatments plans that include exercise, diet, meditation, herbs, yoga, and even massage!

Ayurveda For Beginners

There are plenty of books on Ayurveda on the market, so thanks again for choosing this one! Every effort was made to include all the information you need to introduce you to Ayurveda, and how you can start to incorporate Ayurvedic medicine into your life right now. Please enjoy!

Chapter 1: What is Ayurveda?

Ayurvedic Medicine

You may have heard the term "Ayurveda" before, but have you ever wondered what it really is, where it comes from, and why millions of people rely on it? If so, read on! Ayurveda is a system of medicine that has survived the test of time, and has made great contributions to the alleviation of human suffering. This ancient system of holistic healing has evolved from a rational and logical foundation. The foundation and fundamentals that it's based upon do not change from age to age, making it essentially timeless. Thought to have originated as long ago as 6,000 years BCE, Ayurvedic medicine was recorded in Sanskrit more than 5,000 years ago! This Sanskrit record is found in the Four Sacred Texts called the *Vedas*. These Vedas include the *Sam*, the *Rig*, the *Atharva*, and the *Yajur Vedas*. The Ayurvedic Theory states that every aspect of life impacts our health, and that the *Vedas* cover multiple topics such as health, spirituality, and healthcare, as well as government, astrology, politics, and art. With the medical books of the 8th Century, came procedural instructions based in Ayurveda, as well as how the theory had evolved up to that point in time. It's been said that the true origin of Ayurveda traces all the way back to the Brahmi, the originator of the Universe.

The knowledge we have today is mostly based on what is called the "great triad", which are texts called "*Brhattrayī*", which include the *Charak Samhita, Sushruta Samhita*, and the *Ashtanga Hridaya*.

The Charak Samhita

A major compendium of Ayurvedic medical theory and practice that dates to around 800 BCE. This oldest writing is believed to be one of the most important of authoritative writings on this healing system. The *Charak* is known as a revision of the much older and larger *Agnivesha Samhita*, which is no longer surviving. In the *Charak*, there are more than 8,400 verses that are presented as poetry. Poetry was a way to aid in memorizing information. These 8,400 metrical verses are often committed to memory by modern students of Ayurveda. Focusing on kayachikitsa or internal medicine, the *Charak* is really the first time we see consciousness associated with such consideration and value. It includes discourses on life, being, and at its core, intelligence, and pure knowledge. Even modern physicians of Ayurveda still use the *Samhita* in their training, and rely on multiple translations of the 120 chapters. Charaka was an internist at the University of Taxila, and compiled this text into Sanskrit.

The Sushruta Samhita

A surgical text dating back to 700 BCE. The *Sushruta* includes seminal content such as the definition of health in Ayurveda, as well as information on blood and the description of the five subdoshas of Pitta and marma points. Also included are techniques for skin grafting and reconstructive surgery that led the way. It is thought that this branch of medicine arose party due to the effects of war and that it's a redaction of material passed down verbally through the generations. This *Samhita* is a work of both poetry and prose and is unique, as it's the first to name subdoshas of Pitta. It also considers blood as a fourth doshic principle.

The Ashtanga Sangraha and Astanga Hridaya

These date back to around 400 CE, and were written by a physician of Ayurveda in the Sindh region of India. While the *Sangraha* was originally written in poetry, the *Hridayam* was presented as prose. It's in these two texts that the five subdoshas of Kapha are defined. These three "great" collections of texts were thought to have come along later than the first two, and introduced the Kapha sub-doshas. With this modern organization of the doshas, each of the humors: Kapha, Vata, and Pitta are listed and described. These works highlight treating physiology and provide ideas for the beneficial use of both minerals and metals.

There are other, more minor, classics of Ayurveda. *Sharngadhara Samhita* is an exposition of principles. It's prized for the description of many pharmacological preparations, and it's the first time we see pulse being used as a way to diagnose patients. One of the most recent texts, the *Bhava Prakasha*, is from the 16th Century, and was recently available in English. It contains a re-presentation of the earlier texts, including over 10,000 verses dealing with the characteristics of multiple foods, plants, and minerals. The *Madhava Nldanam* includes classifications of diseases in Ayurveda. From 700 AD, it is valued for going over a wide variety of medical diseases found in women and children, as well as toxicology, and ear/nose/throat diagnoses. There are plenty of educational materials regarding the traditional and historical records of Ayurveda. Dozens of translations and study-guides are available, and if you have an interest in the origins and heart of this practice, I urge you to dive deep into these texts and read the poetry therein.

For example, in Indian philosophy, there are six major schools of orthodox Indian-Hindu philosophy. These include Nyaya, Vaisheshika, Samkhya, Yoga, Mimamsa, and Vedanta. The Samkhya philosophy is the foundation of both yoga and Ayurveda. Samkhya describes how Universal Spirit has changed into physical reality, and clarifies why spirit needs this presence of matter. This explains how our physical world came to become the foundation of other philosophical structures. By establishing a basic dualism between consciousness and matter, it demonstrates a physical world through which that awareness can be experienced or observed. This accounts for why we formed bodies and sensory organs—so our souls can achieve their desire to experience. This philosophy also considers a need of our Souls to rediscover their identity and that every knower requires a "known" to realize itself. With the method that this

Samkhya uses for considering reality, the spiritual sciences of Ayurveda and yoga were formed.

Turning our attention to the philosophical and cultural background that Ayurveda is at its roots, we examine the basic instincts of life. Just as in our cells, those basic instincts include attraction for pleasure and repulsion for pain. It is a study of life as a whole, and it's not exclusively regarding healing the body's ailments. Because of this, there is a vastness and depth to Ayurveda that cannot be grasped or even fathomed with just one reading. It is a practice of theory and application that are meant to be steadily and slowly mastered. This isn't to say that you shouldn't learn about Ayurveda and what it can do in your life. It's a suggestion that you continue learning about Ayurveda in your journey, and that you acknowledge that there is a much deeper understanding regarding the interconnectedness of everything that can only be ascertained through in-depth study. You should experiment by picking up things here and there and practice using medicines and lifestyle changes that relate to your dosha. That will not require anything but a basic knowledge of the fundamental principles. The main one being that ALL living beings are striving to become happy—whether consciously or unconsciously. Its main purpose is to supply all the knowledge necessary to not only maintain health and cure diseases, but to help men to establish a robust outlook in life, thereby proving himself worthy of all the happiness that life has to offer.

The Five Elements

The theory of the five elements, or "Pancha Mahabhuta", according to Charaka, is that each individual is the essence, or embodiment of the universe. In a nutshell, this means that everything existing in the eternity of the Universe is also found in the human body. As a microcosm of it, human beings are a perfect illustration of the universe. The idea that we contain the same elements the universe is translated as the *Panchamahabhutas*. These five "great" elements exist in all matter, and are the building blocks of the universe. These elements manifest and exist in all of nature.

- **Ether/Space**

   Known as "Akasa", ether shouldn't simply be considered the sky. The closest meaning would be "space." Before there was anything, there was nothing. In absolute space where there is nothing, there is neither "here" nor "there." Because space or ether is immeasurable, it is all-pervasive, vast, dimensionless, and essentially, indescribable. In our bodies, all the channels, pores, and empty spaces symbolize akasa. Since it can be challenging to comprehend space, we can think of all the space contained in the cavities of our body: ventricular space, or the cranial cavity, our sinuses, the vertebral cavity, the thoracic cavity, and our abdominal-pelvic cavity.

This ether gives us the space that "allows" for the necessary movement. Think of the space in our brains, or the ventricular space that allows for the passage of cerebrospinal fluid, or the movement of blood in the chambers of the heart. This space exists everywhere—between our cells, within our cells, and even between atoms. Its properties are light, smooth, inactive, soft, clear, neither hot nor cold, separate, and differentiated. Akasa is found in all our body passages and cavities, but is related to the ear. Because of this, it's also related to the sense of sound.

- **Air**

Known as "Vayu", it translates directly as the air. Since space/ether "allows" for the potential to move, if there is no space, then all movement ceases. Air is the principle of movement. With space, there is an inability to measure movement since space itself is immeasurable. From a philosophical perspective, there is a state of being from which the sound "Om" arose, initiating movement via vibration from where the entire Universe came to be. "Va" means "to spread", and it's important to remember that life is movement. This movement is the fundamental function shared by every living organism.

In our bodies, vayu is responsible for various movements, such as electric pulses in our nerves, gastrointestinal movement, joints in motion, etc. Vayu is present in our central nervous system in the form of neurotransmission, motor, and sensory innervation. It's the circulation and movement of our plasma, blood, lymph, and nutrients. It's the ventilation and movement of gases present in all inspired and expired air. Vayu's properties include light, rough, clear, minute, atomic, being neither hot nor cold, and having active movement. It is specifically related to our skin and our sense of touch. The air element provides the driving force behind all movement.

- **Fire**

Known as "Agni", it means "the fire and illumination." As ether evolved into Air, there came space and movement. This movement of Vayu brought with it its vibration. It's the back-and-forth vibrational movement that introduces Agni, since with friction, comes heat. Agni transforms the state of any substance, and is responsible for biotransformation. Agni is active, changeable, and radiant energy. In our bodies, Agni is responsible for biotransforming the food we take in into substances the body can utilize.

Agni's properties include being light, rough, sharp, clear, minute, atomic, hot, dry, luminous, and having a high speed with an active spread. Present in all bodily functions, Agni is related to the eye and our sense of vision. Primary sites are also the liver, stomach, and pancreas. It is typically referred to as the "digestive flame", but should not be limited to the stomach and small intestine. The fire element represents all transformation and illumination. It brings the qualities of attention, appreciation, recognition, ambition, and competitiveness.

- **Water**

Known as "Jala", it translates to "the water." Internally, jala is present in bodily fluids such as blood and spinal fluid, etc. We rely on these fluids to help distribute energy, maintain optimal body temperature, transport hormones, and help with waste elimination. Balancing the heating energy of fire, the cool aspects of water provide the chemical energy that brings molecules together cohesively. Think of condensation—it's any reaction where two molecules combine with the formation and the loss of water. In the evolution of the elements, after the formation of fire through the friction of space and air, water was formed by condensation.

Jala's properties include being heavy, fluid, soft, inactive, slimy, cold, dense, having large molecules, and moving with gravity. The water element is present in all bodily fluids. This includes saliva, plasma, gastric juices, intracellular fluid, urine, stool, and sweat. This element is specifically related to the tongue and our sense of taste. The water element is lubricating, and provides moisture and cooling.

- **Earth**

  Known as "Prithvi", it literally means "earth." This element occurs via solidification, and manifests as physical and mechanical energy. It's seen as the solid support and structure of all matter—both organic and inorganic. Internally, this is represented in our skeleton, cells, and tissues. Prithvi implies steadiness and firmness. Properties include being heavy, rough, hard, slow, inactive, steady, firm, clear, dense, large, bulky, and being neither hot nor cold. Present in our nails, bones, tendons, teeth, muscles, skin, stool, hair, and our spinal cord, Prithvi is directly related to the nose and our sense of smell. The earth element provides structure, stability, and form. The qualities of this element are support, forgiveness, growth, and attachment.

It's these elements and their relations to our sensory organs that work with the three doshas. In this approach to health, there is no distinguishing between "physical" and "mental" aspects. In Ayurveda, before the dosha emerged, the three gunas of nature are what give rise to the five elements. With a basic understanding of the five elements and the three gunas, we can better determine our own constitution when we explore doshas.

The Three Gunas

The gunas are the three basic characteristics or attributes that exist in all things, including our minds and bodies. You will want to explore gunas further in your Ayurvedic journey, but we will go over the psychological aspects since they relate to our moods, emotions, and behaviors. Through an understanding gunas, we can better understand and navigate our internal worlds and work with what life gives us. These three gunas are known as Tamas, Rajas, and Sattva. Everything in nature and all our internal states can be attributed or classified to one of the gunas. Ayurveda shows us how our bodies naturally relate to food, disease, and the environment. It's natural to approach to food is something we don't even think about typically. Through Ayurveda, we can articulate our experiences with food in meaningful ways. It can give meaning and express the therapeutic value of our experiences. This method, the guna method, is an experiential approach in the foundation of Ayurveda. It's simple and practical, so that we can easily grasp the nature of food, what our imbalances are, and what we need to heal.

- **Sattva**

This guna is responsible for all of the goodness of creation, and essentially all of the positive features that make up nature. When we practice Sattvic activities, we permit our minds to be calm and achieve a state of alignment and balance, which takes us to the realization of our true selves. Those that have higher proportions of Sattva are known as healers, teachers, and spiritual leads, as they tend to be wise, noble, and spiritually guided. The spirits of these individuals illuminates their minds, and they can enjoy harmony, balance, peace, and clarity.

Avoiding the other gunas of Tamas and Rajas is essential for gaining and maintaining Sattva. We can also eat Sattvic foods to enhance the guna qualities and to help illuminate our mind. Natural foods such as fruits and vegetables have these qualities. Butter, milk, beans, moderate spices, nuts, grains, and certain herbs are recommended as well. Sattvic states of being include: Delight, happiness, joy, peace, freedom, self-control, satisfaction, cheerfulness, gratitude, fulfillment, trust, empathy, and wellness.

- **Rajas**

This guna is known as the cause behind all activity, and it denotes preservation and passions. Because it expresses itself as a motion, change is in a constant, continuous state. This is also because Rajas is present in all matter. Today's society is filled with those of this Rajasic mindset, and is consumed with negative feelings of ego, domination, and individualization. Those with higher proportions of Rajas are more easily fooled by the concept of "illusion".

This guna is connected with hot, spicy, and heat-inducing foods, because Rajasic actions are typically self-seeking and motivated by a yearning to gain control. This includes foods that are bitter, hot, salty, pungent, dry, and sour. Food items that help enhance the excitement and speed of a person are typically consumed by Rajasic individuals. Rajasic states of being include anger, fear, worry, irritation, as well as determination, rumination, courage, and stress.

- **Tamas**

This is the category of guna associated with delusion, ignorance and the negative attributions stemming from them. In direct opposition to Sattva, Tamas is resistant to the good in nature and resists it, which in turn inhibits the mind from expanding. Violent, hostile, deceitful, and/or immoral actions are considered Tamasic in nature. Characteristics such as vindictiveness, hatred, perversion, and destruction can develop.

Eating processed foods and meats are also included. This also includes liquors, and frozen and/or canned foods as well. These are included because these food items help develop feelings of pessimism and ego. Tamasic states include disgust, laziness, sadness, grief, ignorance, shame, boredom, addiction, dependency, and helplessness.

It is a combination of the three of these gunas that make up the characteristics of all beings. There are many emotions that are found in each of the gunas, so it comes down to the intention or motivation behind any given emotion or action that determines its quality. These gunas make up nature in the same way that the entire spectrum of color can be made from only a few primary colors. When the three of these are in equilibrium, nature is in its purest state, known as "Samyavastha" in Sanskrit. Disruptions in the normal functioning of our bodies are caused when there is an imbalance of these gunas. It is this approach that is referred to as "Ayurveda", and it's grounded in a holistic approach to healing that shows our body as being inseparable from all other environments—spiritual, cultural, or social. The same laws that rule the universe also apply to our bodies.

This means that any and all illnesses come from imbalanced gunas, as it creates conflict to this order. This comes from the idea that the three bodily humors, or doshas, are made up of the five elements. In Ayurveda, when the elements, gunas, and doshas are in balance, there is harmony, longevity, and good health. On the other end of that spectrum, imbalances cause negative effects. Ayurvedic medicine and healing come into play when our health declines or we develop negative effects.

Through promoting the Sattva qualities, Ayurveda aids in restoring balance to the gunas and to clear the mind. In Ayurveda, we can use anything as a form of healing and medicine if used appropriately. The elements can be viewed as a connection that the gunas use to determine the qualities of nature. This also means that imbalances and negative attributes can happen due to the incorrect use of these materials. In Ayurvedic theory, we acquire karmic seeds, or "Daiva", from past lives and the efforts, or "Puruskara", and actions we achieve in our lifetime. In Ayurveda, it's these two concepts of Daiva and Puruskara that pose the fact that we never become ill by chance. It's believed these karmic seeds are responsible for imbalances and poor health. This is the main motive behind Ayurvedic medicine using numerous avenues of healing.

These main systems in therapy are spiritual, psychological, and rational.

- **Rational Therapy** typically directs certain amounts of foods consisting of all natures—Tamasic, Rajasic, and Sattvic. This can be done in conjunction with medication, so that proper balance can be restored to our body.

- **Psychological Therapy** heals our bodies by relying on mind power. It's the interconnectedness of our body and mind that exists in Ayurvedic tradition that makes this method effective. A good way to imagine this is that we cause an imbalance or pain with our thoughts and feelings, and our mind is able to cultivate the needed Sattva to reestablish balance.

- **Spiritual Therapy** will normally involve reciting mantras, fasting, utilizing gemstones, practicing auspicious acts, religious rites, and even sacrifices.

It is through a simultaneous combination of these three main forms of therapy that promotes an efficient healing process between the mind and the amalgamated body. To recap the information we've covered in this chapter, it's through promoting good health and balance that we naturally avoid disease. Many Ayurvedic practitioners believe that everything in the universe is connected, whether it's dead or alive. If we can align our spirit, body, and mind in agreement with the universe, we will have good health, and it's only when something upsets this balance that we become ill. Many things, of course, can upset this balance: Things that we cannot change, such as genetic or birth defects, injuries and age as well as those we can, such as diet, lifestyle, emotions, and climate. Breaking down the word "Ayurveda", we find that it quite literally means the "science of life." "Ayur" literally translates as "life", and "Veda" translates to knowledge or science. Because one of the main principles of Ayurvedic Medicine is that it focuses on the interconnectedness of the mind and body, one of the most powerful ways that we can transform our bodies is through the power of the conscious mind. This means that, through our mental focus, we can begin to change the physical structure of our bodies, and thus, meditation is highly regarded.

Chapter 2: The Three Doshas

In Ayurvedic medicine, there are three governing agents, or "doshas". These are mind-body types that each person can attribute to their unique blend of physical, emotional, and mental qualities. It is also known as the energetic force behind the creation of all physical matter that helps facilitate our mind-body communication. It is important to understand that the Tridosha theory is the dominantideain Ayurvedic medicine. This is the concept that health occurs only when there is a sense of balance of the three senses of humor. Of course, each dosha or humor has its own various physical qualities that govern different aspects of our bodily functions. Because these qualities are always changing and moving, it can cause disruptions when they get out of balance.

As we all have unique fingerprints, we also have patterns of energy. This energy is a distinct blend of our mental, physical, and emotional features which make up our composition. Creating and maintaining a balance of these energies is the main goal in Ayurvedic medicine. By understanding our constitution and the energies that create it, we can take appropriate action to eliminate or minimize the factors that remove us from that balanced state. It is from this balance that we establish and maintain natural order and optimal health. Therefore, the imbalance is illness and disease. We must understand the characteristics and formation of the disorder before the order can be established. These doshas can be used when determining what accounts for the differences in people. Those physiognomies and peculiarities that make each of us unique can be addressed with the doshas.

There are three principles in everything and everyone, and they are related to the biology of our bodies. In Ayurveda, these three basic types of energy do not translate to English as single words, but rather, concepts that we use the original Sanskrit words for still today: Vata, Kapha, and Pitta. To get nutrients and fluids to our cells, movement is required. Energy is essential to creating movement. It is also essential to process nutrients in cells, and is needed to lubricate and maintain the construction of the cell as well. Vata energy is behind all movement, and Pitta is the energy of metabolism and digestion. Kapha is the energy of structure and lubrication. In Ayurveda, the cause of the disease (other than that caused by the presence of toxins) is regarded as an absence of appropriate cellular function due to either a surplus or deficit of one of these three basic types of energy. In every person, there are qualities of all three, but they can be determined as primary, secondary, and third.

Western allopathic medicine (modern, science-based medicine) tends to focus on the symptomatology of the disease and and will primarily use drugs and surgery to prevent and alleviate issues. Because Ayurveda teaches that life must be maintained by balancing energy, they do not focus on the disease itself. While surgery is encompassed by Ayurveda, drugs are considered to weaken the body because of their toxicity. By minimizing anxiety and stress through balancing the movement of energy, the natural defense systems of the body become stronger and can then protect against diseases. That is not to say that we should substitute Ayurveda for modern medicine. There are many times when pharmaceutical drugs and surgery can be the best course of action based on the disease and conditions. It's best to use Ayurveda in conjunction with modern medicine to make us as strong as possible and prevent potential illness, and to rebuild ourselves after being treated with surgery and drugs.

Many times, we may not feel well and we know that something is out of balance, yet when we see a physician, we're advised that nothing is wrong. This is because the imbalance hasn't become a recognizable disease yet. With an Ayurvedic practitioner, they will carefully evaluate the main signs and indications of illness, particularly relative to the causes of an imbalance. Consideration of how suitable various treatments are for an individual is then given. Through direct questioning, observation, and physical examination including monitoring pulse, and by making observations of the eyes and tongue, and in general, our physical form and timbre of our voice, the practitioner can make a diagnosis. To help eliminate an imbalance and manage the cause of the imbalance, palliative (relieving pain without a focus on the cause) care and cleansing measures can be used. Most times, these recommendations include implementing lifestyle and dietary changes. Panchakarma, a five-step rejuvenation experience, is often called for, as well as other cleansing programs to expel toxins and increase the benefit of other treatments.

Vata

Reflecting the elemental qualities of both air and space, Vata translates as "that which moves things." Also known as the "energy of movement", Vata delivers the crucial motion for all our internal bodily functions. These bodily processes rely on motion, as they are crucial for health. With all this moving energy, stabilizing this motion is the main goal of lifestyle adjustments. Finding routines can be very useful for Vata-dominant people, as they typically can grasp concepts quickly, but forget them just as quick. They have quick minds, are flexible, and creative. Those with Vata influence are alert, restless, and very active. They typically will be fast walkers, talkers, and thinkers, but are easily fatigued. Compared to other types, they tend to have less self-assurance, resolution, and tolerance for change, and can often feel ungrounded and unstable. When those with Vata predominance are unbalanced, they can become nervous, fearful and anxious. In Vata, diseases concerning the air principle are more common. These include pneumonia, emphysema, and arthritis. This also includes aching joints, nerve disorders, mental confusion, twitches, as well as dry hair and skin.

Vata dosha-predominance types typically have thin, light, frames and excellent agility. Many of this type will love new experiences and excitement. They can be quick to anger, but they are very quick to forgive as well. When in balance, Vatas take initiative and can be lively conversationalists. The many characteristics of Vata include those that are mobile, subtle and clear. They also include those that are rough, light, cold, and dry, and when in excess, any of these qualities can cause an imbalance. Vata can also be deranged by exposure to cold temperatures and foods, as well as frequent travel (air travel especially) loud noises, over-stimulation, and drugs, alcohol, and sugars. Think of Vata like the wind, where those of this type find becoming and staying grounded difficult. It's important for Vata types to get enough rest, as they need more sleep than the other types. Moisture can be helpful, so steam baths and humidifiers are recommended.

When we have excessive stress in our lives, the Vata force can become imbalanced and our activity can make us start to feel out of control. This can manifest as racing thoughts that lead to anxiety and insomnia. It can also lead to skipping meals, which can result in irregular digestion. If you feel an imbalance, you can adjust your lifestyle to slow yourself down and take your time. Practice meditation, eat regularly-scheduled meals, and get to bed earlier to ensure you get adequate rest. Vata needs to feel grounded and prevented from being carried away. Any choices that bring stability, warmth, and consistency to our lives will help to balance Vata.

Vata Diet

Drawn to those foods that are astringent, such as raw vegetables and salads, they can find balance in foods that are cooked and served warm. They can also be balanced by including the tastes of sour, salty, and sweet. They respond the quickest to warm, moist, slightly oily, and heavy foods. When you are attempting to decrease Vata, you'll want to include warm, well-cooked, unctuous foods. Eating smaller meals three or four times a day is best. Having a routine when it comes to meal times is also important. Digestion can be improved by limiting raw foods and using more oil in the cooking. Again, while keeping away from astringent foods that can be drying, Vata should focus on sweet, ripe, and juicy fruits, as well as well-cooked oats and rice. All dairy products and spices are good, but should be eaten in moderation.

To Balance Vata Energy:

- Rest! Get plenty of sleep
- Create and stick to routines
- Avoid extreme cold, and keep warm
- Avoid stress, and keep calm
- Eat spices and warm foods

Pitta

Pitta types share many qualities of fire, because they carry the energies of both metabolism and digestion. Translated to "that which cooks", the Pitta dosha governs joy, courage, and mental perception. With warm bodies, penetrating ideas and sharp intelligence, Pittas are usually vigilant and have high comprehensive abilities. Pittas are usually of medium height and build with many freckles and moles. They have strong metabolisms, strong appetites, and good digestion. The Pitta constitution can be balanced by astringent, bitter, and sweet tastes. They typically will enjoy hot and spicy foods and cold drinks. Pittas are known for getting sound sleep in moderate amounts. With a lower acceptance for sunlight, physical work, and heat, Pittas sweat easily and have warm extremities. Intelligent and alert, Pittas have great powers of comprehension. Pittas make great leaders and planners, and tend to seek material prosperity and enjoy exhibiting their possessions and wealth.

Diseases that involve fire principles, such as fevers, inflammation, and jaundice, are common for Pitta types. The common attributes for this dosha are: Hot, oily, and mobile. Lifestyle and diet changes should emphasize coolness. Remember that if you're trying to follow a Pitta-pacifying diet, you'll want to pay attention to the generalities and overarching patterns in your current diet. You'll want to gradually shift towards a diet that is more pacifying, rather than trying to follow a strict diet and getting bogged down by details. Find out where you can make small, incremental changes to support you in your healing journey.

When Pitta is in an imbalanced state or in excess, you may find that you sunburn easily. You could be prone to heartburn, diarrhea, anger, agitation, and have flushed nose, cheeks, and/or ears. It can cause aggression and make you easy to anger and experience feelings of jealousy. An imbalance can be caused by being overly competitive, smoking cigarettes, drinking coffee, eating while angry, and by consuming Pitta-aggravating food.

Pitta Diet

Avoid pungent, salty, and sour foods. Refraining from eggs, meat, salt, and alcohol is recommended as well. Incorporating cooling, sweet, and bitter foods and tastes into the Pitta diet will help keep this dosha balanced. Grains such as wheat, rice, and oats are great for reducing Pitta. Stay away from corn, brown rice, and millet. Stick to fruits that include cherries, melons, and oranges that are sweet, while staying away from sour fruits such as berries, and grapefruits. There are plenty of vegetables that will pacify Pitta, such as asparagus, potatoes, broccoli, lettuce, zucchini, and pumpkins. Chicken, turkey, and eggs can aggravate Pitta, so they must be consumed in moderation.

To Balance Pitta Energy:

- Focus on cooling, stabilizing, and sweet
- Balance the amount of activity with rest
- Don't skip meals

- Favor Sweet, bitter, and astringent tastes
- Spend time in nature

Kapha

"That which sticks", the Kapha dosha includes the energies of both construction and lubrication. It is responsible for our physical form, construction, and the smooth operation of all parts. Its characteristics are moist, dull, cold, and static. Associated with the chest, lungs, throat, lymph, fatty tissues, ligaments, and tendons, it can moisten food, build up our tissues, help to store energy, and also lubricate our joints. This dosha governs love, forgiveness, patience, greeting, attachment, and mental inertia. Because it's also associated with the earth, it helps to ground both Pitta and Vata.

While Kapha is nourishing, in excess, it can cause the fluids of the body to flood our tissues. This can cause substantial wetness that can weigh the body down and cloud our minds. A host of disorders such as sinus congestion, obesity, and mucous-related issues thrive in a dense, cold, and swampy environment. When in balance, those of Kapha constitution can be loving and calm, but that turns into lethargy, attachment, and depression in excess. Many Kapha types will have big, soft, eyes and radiant skin. These types tend to sleep well and have steady digestion. They are naturally peaceful, considerate, and loving. Kaphas have an intrinsic ability to relish life, and are contented with routine. In excess, Kapha can be resistant to change and can hold on to things that no longer serve them.

Kapha Diet

It's important to focus on foods that are lighter, drier, and warmer, since Kapha tends to be colder, oilier, and heavier. Foods that are the most beneficial for pacifying Kapha are pungent, bitter, and astringent. You'll want to stay away from the salty, sour, and sweet tastes. Reduce the amount of dairy that you eat as well, since it can increase Kapha. You'll also want to avoid sweeteners while sticking to honey, though in limited qualities. It's recommended that Kaphas with imbalances should make a hot tea with ginger at mealtimes to promote digestion and improve dulled taste buds. All beans can be great food for Kapha other than soybean-based foods. Aim to eat fruits such as pears, apricots, and apples that are light, while avoiding heavy fruits like pineapples, oranges, and bananas.

Almost all spices can pacify Kapha, other than salt. Try pungent spices such as pepper and ginger liberally in your diet. Use only small amounts of fats and oils, and limit the consumption of red meat. Eat lots of vegetables and reduce sweet/juicy vegetables when you can. The Kapha diet needs to include foods that will ignite the metabolic and digestive systems, so it should be dynamic and full of energy. The largest meal should be at lunchtime, and allow at least a few hours after your dinner before going to bed.

To Balance Kapha Energy:

- Seek stimulation
- Find a regular routine
- Stay warm and avoid dampness
- Clear your space/declutter
- Get regular exercise

With any diet to pacify an excess in any certain dosha, you'll want to work on developing your awareness, so that you're continuously inspired to take one small step at a time. Be sure to keep tabs on your health and general sense of well-being, and over time, you'll find that your digestive strength will improve. The goal is to eventually have a diet that supports your capacity to handle more challenging foods with no adverse effects. Work on recognizing the qualities of the foods you love, and those foods that you want to favor in your diet.

Dosha Test

Now that we know the common characteristics of each dosha, it's time to determine which one you are. There are many different Ayurvedic tests online that will help determine your "prakriti", or the constitution that you had at birth. This prakriti consists of the disposition of both your parents, and is responsible for determining your main physical features and emotional behaviors. Of course, online tests or self-led testing will never be perfectly accurate, but they can be used as a guide when observing yourself and deepening your knowledge about your own prakriti.

Any test that you take should be taken at least two or three times, and it's the average of the answers that you'll want to consider to get your dominant dosha. As a basic example of these types of tests, see which of the following you most associate with:

Group A:

- Having a lighter, slimmer physical build and can even be underweight. A thin, angular chin with wrinkled or sunken cheeks. Eyes that are active, small, and dark with a tendency to be dry. Having a nose that is not even, or has a deviated septum. Lips are prone to being dry and cracked while teeth are larger, stuck out and accompanied by thin gums. The skin can be thin and cold as well as rough and dry. Hair as well as nails can be brittle, dark, and dry. The chest and belly can be thin and flat, even sunken in appearance. Hips are slender and the bellybutton can be small or irregular. Internally, joints tend to be cold and cracking. Appetites range, but are irregular and scanty, while digestion tends to cause gas and is usually irregular as well. Preferred tastes are salty, sour, and sweet, and thirst levels change frequently. Mentally, they can be hyperactive and experience emotions of anxiety and uncertainty. They experience insomnia and tend to have sleep issues, with quick and active dreams.

Group B:

- These types have a medium build and weight. With tapering chins and flat cheeks, they will usually have bright and sensitive eyes. Noses can have a red tip, and lips are usually red and inflamed as well. Teeth are medium-sized with tender gums. Overall, skin is oily, rosy, and smooth. Hair is oily and straight, while nails are flexible and sharp. This type usually has very strong appetites, leading to quick digestion. They prefer astringent, bitter, and sweet tastes, and usually have a surplus of thirst. They are prone to feelings of jealousy and anger. They sleep soundly, but experience very little deep sleep and their dreams consist of violence and war.

Group C:

- Heavy and large framed, with a tendency to be overweight. Double chins with rounded, plump cheeks and big, calm eyes are common attributes. They also have button noses with smooth, oil-prone lips. Teeth are healthy and white, with strong gums. Skin tends to be oily and thick as well as hair that is luxuriant. Nails are also oily and smooth, lending to a polished look. Large builds lead to potbellies and big, heavy hips. Joints are typically large, but well lubricated. Appetite can be steady but slow, leading to prolonged digestions and issues with mucous. They prefer tastes that are astringent, pungent, and bitter, and don't get thirsty often. They are slower and more sluggish in eliminating toxins. They get deep, prolonged sleep, and frequently dream of snow, water, and romance.

Which group did you identify most with? If you have a lot in common with Group A, you most resemble the Vata dosha. Group B associates with the Pitta dosha, while Group C is the Kapha dosha. Each of these doshas have attributes and characteristics that can be considered both positive and negative. If you find that you are a "double-dosha" type, remember that these qualities don't blend together, but instead show their influence individually—meaning that either one or the other will present itself at a time. It's possible to be one dosha in mind, and another in the body. Knowing this helps with developing routines for physical and mental issues. Once you've determined your predominate dosha type, begin by creating or following an appropriate diet while practicing lifestyle routines that fit your physical and mental constitution.

The Six Tastes

Another key principle of Ayurveda is a balanced diet that includes eating a wide range of food and spices. It focuses on the six tastes: Sweet, salty, pungent, bitter, astringent, and sour. Depending on your primary dosha, (Vata, Kapha, and/or Pitta) there are specific tastes that will be better suited to your body and what it needs. In Ayurveda, it is incredibly important to taste our foods, and in turn, our lives. Ayurveda views taste, or "Rasa", as a powerful therapeutic tool that can determine not only how we experience the foods we eat, but also the overall flavor of our existence. Because there is a deeper significance, determining the effects that foods, spices, herbs, and experiences have on our state of balance in our body, mind, and spirit is critically important. Each of the six tastes has a role to play in our physiology and health. The endless combination of tastes provides a wide diversity of flavors to encounter. Every detail of a substance should be considered: Where was your food grown or raised? When was it harvested? Was is harvested sustainably? Has it been stored, or preserved? How old or fresh is it? Taste alone can tell us a great deal about the physical and energetic qualities of the food we're taking in. In Ayurveda, taste is a living representation of experience. We should fully acknowledge, appreciate, and even relish all of the flavors we encounter. When we are mindful about these tastes, we can then truly access the potential to affect positive change in our lives.

As we've learned, one of the foundational teachings in Ayurveda is that the five elements make up everything in the universe. This also applies to the six tastes, as each of them contain all five elements, though each is predominantly comprised of two elements.

- **Sweet**

Earth and water elements. A naturally appealing element in our diet, it's the flavor of sugars and many fats, proteins, and carbohydrates. Keep in mind that sweet taste is also in foods that we wouldn't necessarily consider sweet tasting, such as milk and rice. Sweet taste balances both Vata and Pitta, while it can aggravate Kapha. By nature, sweet foods are cooling. The front tip of our tongue is the most sensitive to this taste. Sample foods include bananas, mangos, olives, beets, corn, wheat, navy beans, red lentils, almonds, coconut, beef, pork, basil, tarragon, and all sweeteners.

Sweet taste aids the mucous membranes in our body, including the mouth, lungs, GI tract, urinary tract, and reproductive system. To the mind, sweet taste is strengthening, energizing, nutritive, and soothing. It benefits our skin, hair, and complexion, and aids in the repair of wounds. It can enhance the integrity of the immune system and improves longevity. This is in moderation, however, as an excess of sweetness can smother the digestive fire, diminish appetite, and promote congestion. It also can lead to breathing problems, swollen lymph glands, laziness, fungal infections, obesity, and can contribute to greed and unhealthy cravings.

- **Sour**

Earth and fire Elements. Familiar to us as acids in our foods, we usually associate the sour taste with a watering mouth and a "pucker" from the taste. This taste balances Vata, and can aggravate Pitta and Kapha. By nature, sour taste is heating. On our tongue, sour taste is experienced on the front edges, and along the tapered curve. Sample foods include grapefruit, tamarind, pickles, tomatoes, dough bread, cheese, yogurt, alcohol, vinegar, garlic, and savory foods.

Sour taste fuels the appetite and enhances the secretion of digestive enzymes, stimulating our overall metabolism. It also encourages the flow of bile and promotes good liver function by moving any stagnation found there. It can help awaken the mind and coalesce scattered energy. In excess, this taste can lead to a heightened level of sensitivity in our eyes, ears, and teeth. It can also cause drying of our mucous membranes, cause congestion, acne, excessive thirst, and heartburn. It can also lead to anemia, dizziness, fever, ulcers, and dampness in the lungs. If you have issues with excess heat, congestion, or itching, the sour taste can make it worse.

- **Salty**

Water and fire elements. This taste is derived from salt, and while it aggravates Pitta and Kapha, it balances Vata. In temperature, it's mildly heating. On the tongue, the rear edges are sensitive to this taste. Foods would include celery, seaweed, cottage cheese, tuna, any form of salt, soy sauce, and tamari. Because it increases salivation, it supports digestion, absorption, assimilation, and elimination. It helps us maintain our water-electrolyte balance, promotes growth, supports muscle strength, and moistens the body. Salty taste can be soothing to our nervous systems and even help guard against tumors. Using it as an enhancing agent, it can help combat dullness, depression and a lack of creativity. In moderation, it is nourishing to the plasma, prevents stiffness, and enhances the spirit.

In excess, the salty taste will overshadow all other flavors completely. It's important to balance this taste, as it can disturb all of the other doshas. Too much can cause water retention, leading to viscous blood and high blood pressure. Excess can also hinder sensory perception, cause bleeding disorders, infertility, and aggravate skin conditions.

- **Pungent**

Fire and air Elements. Found in many spicy foods, herbs, and spices, the pungent taste is one of dry heat. Usually found in the presence of resins and aromatic volatile oils, it stimulates the tissues and nerve endings of the mouth with a sensation of heat. It balances Kapha, while aggravating Pitta and Vata. The central region of the tongue is sensitive to the pungent taste. Foods include garlic, leeks, turnips, spelt, mustard seeds, pepper, most spices, ginger, and paprika. This taste warms the body, clarifies the sense organs, and cleanses the mouth. It's known to kindle the digestive fire, improve digestion, absorption, and elimination. When balancing excess Kapha, the pungent taste is crucial, as it can support the elimination of excess fat. It's stimulating, penetrating, and clears congestion, moisture, and stagnation. The pungent taste also aids in circulation, clears toxins, cleans the blood and muscles, and opens the internal channels.

In excess, the Pungent taste can be very drying and can lead to giddiness, tremors, insomnia, and muscle pain. An excess can lead to sexual debility in both sexes. It can cause burning, fainting, bleeding, heartburn, constipation, and nausea. In excess, the pungent taste can even be carcinogenic, causing mental confusion, depression, malaise, and debility.

- **Bitter**

Air and ether elements. Another familiar taste, most people avoid it, though some enjoy it. Its temperature is cooling, and it balances Pitta and Kapha, but can aggravate Vata. The middle edges on both sides of our tongue are sensitive to this taste, as well as a small band across the middle of the tongue. Foods include burdock root, kale, eggplant, bitter melon, sesame seeds, coffee, dark chocolate, cumin, saffron, and turmeric. Because it scrapes fats and toxins from the body, the bitter taste is deeply cleansing. While improving other tastes, it also stimulates a healthy appetite. It alleviates thirst, kills germs, and can clear parasites from the GI tract. The bitter taste can tone the muscles and skin, relieve gas, reduce fainting tendencies, and eliminate excess moisture from the body.

In excess, this taste can induce nausea, cause dry mouth, deplete the tissues, and weaken the lungs and kidneys. Too much bitter taste can cause malaise, confusion, coldness, and even loss of consciousness.

- **Astringent**

Air and earth elements. This is a flavor of dryness that is produced by tannins in the bark, leaves and outer fruit rinds of trees. The astringent taste causes mucous membranes to contract, and produces a drying sensation in the mouth. It balances Pitta and Kapha, while aggravating Vata. It's cooling, and is sensitive to the central region on the back of the tongue. This taste absorbs moisture and cleanses the mucous membranes.

It promotes the clotting of blood, scrapes fat, and improves absorption.

Foods include apples, pomegranates, avocados, green beans, potatoes, rye, beans, popcorn, chicken and venison, basil, saffron, and rosemary. The binding effects of the astringent taste can tone loose and flaccid tissues and correct sinking imbalances. It can also improve wound healing and avert coughs. In excess, it can create dry mouth, choking, bloating, and constipation. It can even cause emaciation, convulsions, and stroke paralysis.

There are other influences regarding the foods we eat. We start with taste that is either single or a combination of the six tastes. We then consider whether the food is pacifying or aggravating on each of the doshas. We also want to consider whether the food or substance is heating or cooling in nature, by assessing its temperature, or "Virya". Even further, we look at the post-digestive effect, or "Vipka", to determine the effects and nourishment given to individual cells. Another part of this complex set of influences is the "Prabhava", or the unpredictable action(s) that are unique to a substance. For example, ghee has a cooling effect, yet it also kindles the digestive fire. Of course, we look at the associated qualities, or gunas. From there, we consider any affinity for tissues and/or organs, the direction of movement within the body, and any emotional influence.

It's the combination of all these factors that affect a wide range of responses in each person. Every substance is unique, but each of the six tastes will exert a predictable influence on our physiology.

Chapter 3: Healing Using Ayurvedic Theory

Yoga

While Ayurveda is the science of health, yoga is the actual practice of this science. These are two disciplines that need to be studied and practiced close together. Yoga has no curative aspects by itself, as it focuses on psychological methods and physical strength. It's with Ayurveda that you complete the system in terms of diet, lifestyle, and curative aspects of health. The three universal energies, or "Gunas", are Sattva, Rajas, and Tamas. These represent calm, passion, and inertia, and they are harnessed in all yogic practices that have the goal of energizing us and bringing us to a state of peace. Ayurvedic medicine in practice typically prescribes dietary advice as well as yogic practices that will be most beneficial to a person'sbody type. It's acceptable to think of them as the same disciplines of a larger system of health. As mentioned in Chapter 1, the philosophical system Samkhya Darshan is at the basis of both yoga and Ayurveda. This Samkhya is a complete metaphysical system that explains the manifestation of the world from pure consciousness, all the way down to the five elements. Both Ayurveda and yoga are arts in balancing these five elements within each of us to achieve optimum health and emotional balance.

Ayurveda For Beginners

These "sister sciences" have developed together and have influenced each other heavily throughout history. They show us how to understand the language of nature and of life, so that we can live in harmony within the universe. As we heal the individual, we heal the community and society. Together, yoga and Ayurveda are a complete discipline that can transform our existence from merely physical to the deepest spiritual levels of our beings. Traditionally, yoga deals with our spiritual aspects in life, while Ayurveda deals with mental and physical disease and the adjustments we can make to our lifestyle regimens. Yoga was prescribed as exercise, or physical therapy, in theory and in application. Because this physical side of Ayurvedic healing is only part of the whole system, it's recommended that you practice the inner aspect of healing the subtle body and the mind through yoga as well.

So how do you know what type of yoga is best for you? Take your "Vikruti", or imbalance, into consideration. This is the most important aspectof your regime since we can stay in good health once we are in balance by finding yogic poses that balance "Prakruti", or your constitution. For those of Vata dosha constitution, you will find that you are most braced by practices found to be warming, quieting, and those that are calming. For those of Pitta predominant dosha, that would mean calming, quieting, and cooling. Kapha dosha constitutions will be best supported by a warming and stimulating yoga practice. If you are practicing yoga in ways that do not support you, you are inviting greater imbalance. Below are a few "Asanas", or yoga postures, for each dosha type. Keep in mind that these are overly simplistic explanations of each pose, and you should consider your constitution as well as your age, the time of day, and the season you are in while practicing. Find a yoga practice in your area, and take a test class if you've never tried it before. You should find that they are very welcoming, and look forward to helping you on your healing journey.

Vata Asanas

Calming and grounding asanas are most suitable for Vata dosha types, as they will help you avoid the tendency to be nervous, restless, and being "spaced out." They help alleviate worry and fear and realign physical balance disparities such as joint pains, back pains, and constipation known to accompany Vata imbalances. Because the intestines, pelvis, and lower abdomen are the main residences for this dosha, these asanas work to compress and tauten the lower abdomen while strengthening the lower back. Keep in mind that most asanas are great for harmonizing Vata, because the majority of them help to calm the mind.

- **Uttanasana/Standing Forward Bend**
  One of the best asanas for Vata, you begin by standing with feet a shoulder-width away from each other. Hands and arms can be raised above the head or bent at the elbows holding the opposite arm, while allowing the forearms to relax on top

of the head. While maintaining a straight back, bend forward from your hips slowly while exhaling, and stretch as far frontward as is comfortable. You may keep your hands crisscrossed, or simply rest them on the floor in front of the feet, or clasp them behind your heels if you can. If you aren't as flexible, you can use blocks or books. Allow gravity to aid in lengthening your spine. This is a standing asana and it is used as a grounding technique when awareness is drawn to the feet, where you honor the linking between your physical body and the earth. If you are suffering from a tight back, this asana should work wonderfully for you. If you have limitations, you can always perform the pose while sitting, known as "Paschimottanasana".

- **Balasana/Child's Pose**
  This asana is great for compressing the pelvis, and for relieving constipation and chronic gas. Sitting up straight with your knees underneath your bottom, arms should be at your sides. You move forward, advancing from your hips until you can place your head on the floor. Try using a pillow or a folded blanket on the floor if you can't reach it.

- **Supta Virasana/ Hero Pose (Reclining)**
  Another great pose for Vata, this pose begins with kneeling with our knees together and our bottoms sitting on our heels.

Push your legs to the side of your pelvis, so your bottom is able to go down between your legs. You then put your hands on the bottoms of your feet and stretch back onto your elbows. This can be a tough stretch for most of us, so just work on gradually lowering the back as near to the floor as you can. You can keep the hands by your side, or you can stretch them overhead to help extend the spine.

Pitta Asanas

Calming and cooling asanas are most suitable for Pitta dosha types, as calming poses will help to sedate the intensity that is common for them. These poses are great as a component of treatment for ulcers, liver disease, acne, and hyperacidity. To balance Pitta, these asanas work by placing weight on the solar plexus region and the navel. They affect our spleen and liver by helping to regulate the strength of the digestive fire.

- **Ustrasana/Camel Pose**
  This asana helps to open the abdomen, chest, and solar plexus and allows for a greater flow of energy around these areas. Begin by standing up on your knees. Place palms on your bottom and move your pelvis and thighs forward while you stretch your lower back and bring your hands to the top of your heels. Stretch your neck gently and breathe mindfully.

- **Bhujangasana/Cobra Pose**

  Lying down on your stomach with legs together and ankles stretched out, you bend the elbows and put your hands on the floor by your upper stomach. You can also place your palms at shoulder level if you are less flexible. As you breathe in, extend your elbows while raising the abdomen (and head and chest) off of the floor. Keep your pelvic bones on the floor and hold your head in a neutral or extended position.

Kapha Asanas

Asanas that are heating and more stimulating are called for when balancing the cold, slow, heavy, and sedated nature of Kapha. Asanas that open up the chest are ideal, as Kapha accumulates in the chest and stomach. The following asanas help to prevent and treat congestive and constrictive conditions. The sedating and calming effect of asanas should be balanced out by poses that are heating and stimulating. Kapha dosha types are well-matched to handle strengthening poses, and they should work on increasing flexibility, as it's easy for this type to become overly stiff or rigid.

- **Setu Bandha/Bridge Pose**

  Lying on our back, arms at our sides and palms down towards the floor, we use our elbows and forearms to raise our pelvis off of the mat as we keep our shoulders and feet grounded. Focus on staying on your shoulders and work to raise the pelvis by extending through both of your legs. You can modify this by laying over a pillow. This asana will open the chest and allow for increased circulation of energy. This also affects the flow of energy through our heart chakras, which will aid in the development of unconditional love and compassion.

- **Suryanamaskar/Sun Salutation**

  Obesity and depression are common Kapha conditions, and this asana is a great aerobic exercise as it will get your blood pumping while raising your temperature and expanding your chest. Kapha dosha types should perform many repetitions of this asana, and perform them with great speed. Sun salutations can benefit all constitutions, especially during Kapha dominant energy timings—6:00-10 a.m. and p.m. Standing erect with feet touching, elbows bent with hands together in the middle of the chest, you raise your arms up and stretch into a backbend. You then lean forward and put the hands on the floor, remembering to bend your knees if needed. From this pose, you move backward with your right leg while bending your left knee. You can rest the other knee on the floor and keep the foot of your left leg between your hands. You then bring your left leg backward, next to the right leg as you move into the pose Downward-Facing Dog. Bring your elbows down to the floor and move your body

into the Cobra Pose. You then move back into the
Downward-Facing Dog. Then, move your right leg forward
as you return, and then stand while raising the arms over your
head again. To finish the cycle, you bring your hands to your
chest with palms together.

Ayurvedic yoga is unique in its style because you're using the
understanding of your body and lifestyle to find the appropriate
asanas. Poses are chosen individually to balance your unique
imbalances, and this leads us to attain a higher level of wellness as
compared to other yoga styles. Practicing yoga through Ayurveda
can help eliminate sleep issues, reduce stress, help one lose weight,
balance hormones, reduce illness and disease, keep the mind/body
balanced, and minimize inflammation due to health-related issues.

Chakras

Chakras, or "wheel/vortex" in Sanskrit, are seven points that can be
"tapped" into for increased health, vitality, and greater spiritual and
mental powers. Ayurvedic practitioners use these energies to
describe disease to balance the energy in the body. When out of
balance, we experience many health and relationship issues. When in
balance, it can lead to harmony, prosperity, and higher
mental/spiritual powers. It's important to understand that chakras

are contained within the subtle energy body, and are connected through a central channel. Picture this as a broad, white band to the front of your spinal column, running from the root to the crown chakra. By working on balancing each chakra, or by focusing on moving energy up and down the central channel, we can promote the health of our body, mind, and spirit.

While exploring Ayurvedic medicine, you'll find aligning and maintaining the balance of chakras is a key practice. Our cerebrospinal system has over 72,000 nerves, and is the power supply system for our bodies. Think of the chakras as the main switchboards of this power system. How does one balance the chakras? There are many techniques that we can employ to create balance within the chakras. They include meditation, self-reflection, reiki, holistic medicines, breathing exercises, and other forms of therapy. There is also the practice of cleaning and healing our chakras as well. This is where we restore the balance of the energy levels of the collection of chakras.

Below is a breakdown of the seven chakras:

- **Sahasrara/Crown (7)**

  Associated with no color, or the color white. This chakra is present in our crown and symbolizes self-actualization, spirituality, and oneness. This energy center is the straight connection we have to the universe. It governs spirituality, cohabitation, harmony, and unity with all life. The crown chakra is all about feeling blissful energy and knowing how to communicate with it to uplift the consciousness of humanity. When this chakra is out of balance, we may experience headaches, mental illness, senility, feeling stuck mentally, worry, and a lack of faith or belief.

To balance and open this chakra, we should find ways to create a link between ourselves and the spiritual world. Start a vision board or dream journal to discern intentions in a sacred space. Try guided visualization meditations involving light coming into your head and filling you with energy. Eat violet and white colored foods, and practice meditation using gemstones such as fluorite and amethyst. Exercises that use the Lotus Position can be beneficial for pushing energy through this chakra.

- **Ajna/Third Eye (6)**
  Associated with the color indigo, and the "Tattva" or reality/truth element, this chakra is present in the space between our eyebrows, and signifies self-realization. It also signifies the distinction between men and divine consciousness, and provides knowledge about sight and intuition, as well as inner vision. Home to our spiritual and instinctive sense, the sixth energy center is associated with imagination, instinct, awareness, and clearness. When

balanced and opened, this third eye energy center allows us to clearly see circumstances and overcome the anguish that arises with misinterpretations. It's connected to the psychic and telepathic capabilities that direct us to this universal wisdom. Imbalances can be represented by poor memory, confusion, fogginess, inability to concentrate, sleep disorders, and psychic misinterpretations.

Meditating with the intention of focusing the mind is a great way to begin when balancing the third eye chakra. Try to meditate in the outdoors in sunlight or moonlight. Get enough sleep to promote clear thinking and improve dream recollections. Find indigo-colored foods like figs and blackcurrants to enhance this chakra's function. Eat foods like kale and seaweed, since the calcification-prone pineal gland is a large component of this chakra. Find indigo gemstones like sodalite and azurite. Wear deep-blue-colored clothing, and try to surround yourself with this color. Find exercises that stimulate your temples and meditations that visualize the energy of the sun.

- **Vishuddha/Throat (5)**

Associated with blue, and the void or space/ether element, this chakra is located at our throat, and is responsible for the sense of truth that we have. It suggests our spiritual awakenings, the power of communication, attentiveness, as well as logic and reason. Defining our expressive capabilities, the throat chakra is connected to our personal voice and truth. Blockages in this chakra can manifest when we do not let our emotions out in healthy ways. If we do not express how we truly feel inside, we can create great imbalances in this chakra, leading to a thin, hoarse voice, and stuffiness and itchiness in our throat. Other signs of imbalance include anxiety, stuttering, jaw stiffness, thyroid imbalances, fevers and flu, and swollen glands.

Because this chakra relates to our expression, we should try to focus openness to our throats by singing, reciting poetry, and by having meaningful conversations where we can express our emotions and inner thoughts. Find gemstones such as aquamarine and amazonite to meditate with. Focus on exercises that strengthen the thyroid.

- **Anahata/Heart (4)**
  Associated with green, and the air element. At the center of our chest and spine, this chakra indicates love, devotion, compassion, and transformation. The heart chakra ensures our capability of expressing our love and emotion for each other. It also helps fulfill the gap between our lower and higher energies.When in harmony, this chakra helps us step into the world with loving hearts and open minds. It inspires integrity and ethical conduct, and a joining to others through

our hearts and minds. This chakra is closely linked to our mindful and personal self as opposed to our physical being. As it is also related to emotions, it can be tough to preserve a balanced and opened heart chakra when we are upset, negative, stressed, or hurt. When imbalanced, we can experience muscular tension, chest pain, passivity, heart disorders, breathing trouble, and passivity.

We can balance our heart chakras by inviting more energy of pure love into our bodies. Go on walks and spend time with loved ones, or spend time helping others. Be active in your compassion to charge this chakra, and help it to feel full. Eat green foods like spinach, limes, and greens. Find gemstones such as emeralds to use in meditation, or to place around your home. Find ways to wear green and surround yourself with nature and the outdoors. Focus on exercises that expand the chest and strengthen the lungs.

- **Manipura/Solar Plexus (3)**
  Associated with yellow, and fire energy, the solar plexus chakra is located above our navel and ensures the presence of self-worth, power, and bodily functions. It also is related to our appearance, responsibilities, and proper sensitivity within us. It's through this third chakra that we gain self-confidence, good digestion, and emotional balance. It propels us forward to fulfill our dreams and goals. When fully stimulated, we are

more mindful to our purpose in life, and the course we wish to live our lives. Inspiring creativity that can be expressed through art, home, music, work, and relationships, the solar plexus chakra helps us to preserve a robust personal character. It creates a balance between personal enablement and concern. When out of balance, we can experience indigestion, self-shame, gallstones, pancreatic and liver problems, and adopt an overachiever personality.

Explore art classes, doing puzzles, and reading empowering books to balance your solar plexus chakra. You can remove stagnancy, thereby inviting creativity and following through with tasks. Get out in the sunshine and find detoxification programs that can help with digestion. Find ways to incorporate yellow foods like squash and lemons, and teas like chamomile to boost this chakra's energy. Find yellow gemstones like citrine. Wear yellow, and look for essential oils containing lemon and rosemary. Look for exercises that strengthen your stomach.

- **Svadhishthana/Sacral (2)**
  Associated with orange and the water element, our sacral chakra is related to the well-being of our sexuality, vitality, and desire for love. It is also related to sensuality, emotional interactions, and relationships. Known as being the "boiler room" of our energy system, the sacral chakra assists us in

being hands-on and self-assured in life. This is the chakra involved in experiencing birth and creativity, and even sexuality. It provides a feeling of strength and wellness in terms of overall health, and provides grounding, centeredness, and stabilization. When we have an imbalance of the sacral chakra, we can experience asthma and allergies, depression, eating disorders, impotence, dulled senses, and even urinary problems.

When balancing your sacral chakra, you'll want to get out and relax by the open water. This provides relaxation for emotions, as well as increases the chakra's energy flow. Swimming and other physical activities that take place in a natural setting such as lakes or the ocean are ideal. Join a water aerobics class, watch rainstorms, and find ways to surround yourself with open water. Eat orange-colored foods such as oranges, sweet potatoes, and carrots. Practice meditation using orange gemstones like amber and tiger's eye, or place these stones around your home. Balance this chakra by surrounding yourself with orange. Find exercises that focus on strengthening the kidneys and the abdomen.

- **Muladhara/Root (1)**
  Associated with red, and the earth element, this chakra is positioned at the bottom of our spine. The root energy center looks after our connection with the earth and helps us

to feel grounded, as well as promoting our instincts. Known as being the house of the unconscious mind, this chakra provides the drive for survival, instincts, and basic needs. When this chakra is in balance and is healthy, you're more likely to practice good habits of self-care. It can help us to feel inspired and trust all aspects of our lives. It helps us to feel like we're being taken care of, and even that we know how to handle money responsibly. When we are experiencing an imbalance of the root chakra, we can experience fatigue, poor circulation, cold hands and feet, back pain, anemia, and frequent colds.

To balance your root chakra, you'll want to practice physical exercise and getting sound sleep. Look for activities that connect you with earthy energy, such as gardening or pottery. Try to incorporate red foods and teas into your diet. Use red gemstones in meditation practices or place them around your home to boost the energy of this chakra. You can increase this energy as well by wearing red clothing, bathing with red oils, and surrounding yourself with red flowers. Find exercises that stimulate the perineum and sphincter muscle.

When our chakras are cleansed, healed, and balanced, we will know by the equilibrium of our energy. We can tell by feeling the different and distinct qualities of each chakra. We will feel an appropriate intensity and energy level of each chakra. We can feel the appropriate direction of the chakras, as well as the polarity and flow. With practice and experience, you will feel if anything is off. You can then take the steps necessary to heal them and lead an active lifestyle with more balance. Expand your knowledge through meditation. Explore and create an awareness and understanding with each energy center, so that you can allow yourself to embody the qualities of each chakra.

Aromatherapy

Ancient aromatherapy included burning various woods, and included the use of smoke. Using aromatics for medicinal, cosmetic, and odor-absorbing purposes goes back thousands of years. Ayurvedic physicians or "Vaidyas", treated the royalty with herbs, flowered waters, and aromatic oil massages. Aromatherapy is considered an important tool in Ayurveda regarding prevention and healing. It's used to protect the vital force, or "Prana". It's used to regulate digestion and metabolism, or "Agni". Some practices in Ayurveda involve smoke therapy. An example of this would include burning neem leaves, and burning incense while meditating. Some Ayurvedic practices mix different scents into combinations that intensify strength, and balance the overall effect.

Through our sense of smell, vapors stimulate our olfactory nerves. Because the olfactory nerves arouse the limbic system, we can use aromatherapy to influence everything from emotions, desires, appetites, memories, and even stimulate the endocrine glands to regulate our hormones. An aromatherapy massage is also widely used as a healing technique in Ayurveda. Through massage, we inhale the essential oils as well as absorb them through our skin. By penetrating the tissues, these oils are taken up by the bloodstream and then transported to our systems. This method can be especially beneficial when balancing the dosha or adjusting your body to seasons. Aromatic baths are also popular, as the surface of the water instantly vaporizes the oils and sends the particles to our brain. While we receive the benefit of soaking and relaxing our muscles, we enhance the effect of the aromas. There are various applications to aromatherapy, and it's easy to find ways to incorporate this practice into your lifestyle.

We can balance our doshas with aromatherapy, and promote overall healing as well. Below, we'll explore Ayurvedic aromatherapy for each dosha.

- **Vata**

  When too much air has accumulated in our mind, body, and environment, we experience an imbalance of Vata. This can express itself as a feeling of not being grounded, and we can balance this by bringing more earth and stability into our physiology. Oils must be damp, soothing, and warm. Look for oils such as bergamot, lemon, orange, ginger, and cardamom. Floral scents such as geranium and rose are also calming and can help with sleep problems that are common for Vatas. Sweet citrus scents can help balance energy. For massage, look for carrier oils such as sesame, castor, and avocado oils. When shopping or creating your essential oil to balance Vata energy, look for complex blends that include up to eight oils to find the right combination for optimum balance.

- **Pitta**

  When too much fire has accumulated, our Pitta is out of balance. This results in a sense of external and internal combustion. By bringing in more space and coolness to our physiology, we can balance excess Pitta. Pitta types are typically intense and passionate, and there is often a need to cool, clarify, and ease the mind. Ideal scents include astringent, bitter, and sweet. Look for oils that have a cooling and drying effect, and those that allow excessive heat to escape from the body. These types of oils include sandalwood, lavender, fennel, sandalwood, and ylang ylang. Because Pittas can be very visual, it's important to incorporate live flowers in their living and meditation spaces. Carrier oils such as olive, almond, and sunflower are ideal.

Try a bath infusion of ylang ylang and sandalwood on hot days.

- **Kapha**

  When we feel sluggish, congested, and dull, it can be a sign that too much earth has accumulated in our mind, body, and environment. A Kapha imbalance can be corrected by bringing more movement and circulation into our lives, or invigoration. Because Kapha types are heavy and solid, leading to depression and sluggishness, we should look for oils that are light, warm, and dry. Look for pungent, stimulating scents such as sage, cedar, pine, and basil. Scents such as peppermint can be stimulating and increase motivation physically. Look for oils such as anise, clary sage, tea tree, grapefruit, and camphor. As Kaphas can be moist and oily by nature, they may have trouble absorbing additional oil in significant quantities. Use carrier oils such as grapeseed, almond, and mustard seed.

Because essential oils are so potent, it's extremely important that you extend great care in blending and using them. Always mix oils in a carrier oil or in water, and never apply essential oils directly to your skin. You'll want to test all oils for your levels of sensitivity, and it's wise to consult your physician before starting on any aromatherapy program. This is extremely important if pregnant, nursing, or if there are existing conditions.

Ayurvedic Herbal Remedies

In addition to lifestyle changes and dietary recommendations, Ayurveda also includes many herbal blends for healing. There are more than 5,000 herbs used in this traditional system of healing, and many are well-suited for resolving common problems that we experience today. Many of these herbs have similar mechanisms of action, and they each have unique qualities.

Let's explore some of the more common herbal remedies in Ayurveda:

- **Ashwagandha**

  Indicated for stress, anxiety, and adrenal dysfunction, this herb can also be an alternative to antidepressant and anti-anxiety medications. Ashwagandha has been known to lower our levels of stress hormone, cortisol, and can enhance our natural levels of testosterone and DHEA-hormones that help maintain our strength and muscle mass. This herb is also used to calm inflammation. Known for being an adaptogen, this herb assists us to deal with stress by decreasing blood sugar and by increasing brain function. Ayurvedic practitioners have used ashwagandha, or "smell of the horse" in Sanskrit, for improving concentration, as well as energy levels. Considered a safe supplement for most people, it's still recommended that you consult your physician before supplementing with this herb. When used correctly, ashwagandha can be an easy and effective way to improve your health and overall quality of life. In a nutshell, ashwagandha is revered because it promotes energy and stamina without stimulating the heart.

- **Arjuna**

  Widely used in Ayurvedic medicine, arjuna is used to control hypertension and other cardiovascular ailments. Also known for treating asthma and kidney stones, arjuna, or "shining" in Sanskrit, also contains several substances that produce a strong antioxidant effect. This herb is known to support the heart's energy output and increase overall energy levels, stamina, and immunity. It also helps reduce and relieve mental stress and nervousness. This herb has shown to interact with free radicals and stabilize them and can even lower our levels of bad cholesterol while enhancing our good cholesterol! Commonly used as a supplement or tincture, arjuna is created using the bark from the arjuna tree. As the heart is the one organ that receives all of the stress signals of the body, it's important that we take special care of our hearts. Arjuna has been used historically to support the heart's lymph drainage, and encourage healthy muscular contractions.

- **Curcumin**

A true treasure in Ayurveda, curcumin is one of the main components of the turmeric plant. Known for enhancing flexibility and joint integrity, it's a powerful natural remedy for chronic inflammation. Curcumin is the main health-promoting component of the turmeric plant. In supplements, curcumin is concentrated to work more quickly than the whole root. While incorporating turmeric into your daily dietary plan is advisable, if you're seeing relief for something immediate, you'll want to take curcumin. Used for its anti-inflammatory effects, curcumin can also suppress inflammation without gastric complications. Turmeric and curcumin are powerful antioxidants, and can increase vitamin E in plasma levels after just a few months of regular use.

- **Triphala**

One of the classic combinations of Ayurvedic herbs, triphala includes haritaki, bahera, and amla. This blend is used to enhance digestion and regularity, and for helping good bacteria to flourish in the gut. Often used as a mild laxative, this herbal concoction has been used for thousands of years in Ayurveda. Triphala includes sweet, astringent, bitter, pungent, and sour tastes. When taken nightly, it's common to notice various flavors and tastes every time. The theory behind this is that you're missing from your diet whatever it is your taste. Using this data, it's easier to create your meals and integrate suitable tastes to create balance. You shouldn't taste

sweetness often, as it indicates that you should stop
consuming triphala.

- o Haritaki—This herb alone has a laxative effect, as well
as having an anti-diarrheal effect. Known for being
anti-inflammatory and calming to Vata energy,
haritaki is believed to have multiple positive effects
on the brain and the heart. Buddha is usually
depicted extending a handful of the haritaki fruit—
indicating its longstanding medicinal use.
- o Bahera—A powerful rejuvenator that has detoxifying
qualities on our blood, muscles, and fatty tissues.
This herb is extremely useful in conditions that
involve excess mucous, and is good for quality bone
formation. This fruit is known as the one who keeps
away disease, and it has multiple effects on Kapha.
- o Amla—The Indian gooseberry is also a prized
rejuvenator in Ayurveda. Amla is known for lowering
cholesterol, and contains high amounts of vitamin C.
This fruit is great for balancing Pitta.

For beginners, it is advised that you start with
standardized capsules taken before each meal. When
taken consistently, you can see results within two weeks,

though you should allow up to six weeks for the full therapeutic effect.

- **Trikatu**

  Known as "three peppers" or "pungent", this is a complementary formula to triphala. The combinations of peppers have effects in the upper GI tract, where it enhances the digestive fire. Consisting of black pepper, Indian long pepper, and ginger, Ayurvedic practitioners recommend trikatu as a warming formula to awaken digestion and destroy accumulated waste and toxins. It is also used to enhance the bioavailability of drugs, nutrients, and to increase digestive enzymes. Also recommended to be taken before meals, its best taken in capsule form.

- **Holy Basil**

  A traditional Ayurvedic remedy for colds and flu, holy basil, or "tulsi", helps relieve respiratory infections and seasonal allergies. Typically found in a combination of herbal formulas, holy basil is considered sacred by many in India. Found growing in temple gardens, the rich fragrance helps open respiratory passages, and according to some, helps the spirit soar. Similar to the active compounds in oregano, tulsi shares their anti-inflammatory and analgesic actions. The compounds found in the oil of this herb show antimicrobial and antifungal properties. Originally used as an anti-tussive in classical Ayurveda, it clears excess dampness in the lungs. Holy basil can also reduce stress in those that suffer from generalized anxiety disorders. Available in supplements and great for teas, tulsi is an excellent way to incorporate Ayurvedic herbal healing into your daily routine.

- **Neem**

Neem is known as "the wonder tree" in Ayurvedic medicine, because it's a power plant that can clean and purify the blood and support skin and overall health. Because the skin is our largest organ, it works hard to regulate our temperature while protecting everything it contains. It can also be a clear indication of our internal health. Neem oil is growing in popularity in the West, as it's an overall detoxifier and flushes toxins out through the sweat glands. Being useful in preventing and treating shingles and nerve pain, neem is also used in treating ringworm. It can lower blood sugar levels and must be taken with food. It's a strong remedy for fungal, bacterial, and viral infections.

- **Dashamoola**

An herbal formulation that combines the health benefits of different medicinal plants. These plants' roots are combined in equal amounts to make this ancient Ayurvedic remedy: Bilva, agnimantha, brihati, gambhari, kantakari, gokshura, patala, shalaparni, prishniparni, and shyonaka. These plant roots in combination have antioxidant, painkilling,

74

detoxifying, and anti-inflammatory properties that are used to ease symptoms and tackle multiple ailments where they start. Some of the multiple benefits of this formulation are outlined below:

- o A tonic for the lungs, dashamoola helps to soothe a dry cough and make it easier to breathe. A formulation was given to asthmatics to alleviate symptoms, and it's a known remedy for whooping cough.

- o Because it has antipyretic properties, Ayurvedic practitioners use dashamoola to treat high fevers. It can be used to help bring down a fever and make one feel better since it can help one feel less fatigue.

- o It can help ease symptoms of migraines and recurrent headaches. Known to improve symptoms of nausea and gastrointestinal issues, it also eases light sensitivity, pain around the eyes, and acidity in the stomach. Administered through nasal oil, this can be a powerful headache reliever.

- o Dashamoola can be administered as an enema to help overcome Vata food allergies and relieve built-up gas.

o One of the most popular uses for dashamoola is in the treatment of inflammatory disorders and pain-relieving effects. This is important for those that suffer from arthritis, or other inflammatory issues associated with pain.

o For females with menstrual issues, dashamoola can help. It's been known to relieve lower back pain, anxiety, mood swings, and insomnia. As an herbal tea, it can help with premenstrual syndrome and issues throughout the cycle.

Mantras

At the most refined level, everything in creation is sound or vibration. Everything has its own unique vibration, even the qualities in our life such as joy and love. When we are happy and healthy, these vibrations harmonize with each other. If these vibrations become distorted, this harmony breaks down, and we can experience discomfort and a lack of wholeness. Ayurveda practitioners practice healing through mantras, as a way to restore balance, harmony, and create comfort. These mantras are specific sounds and/or vibrations whose effects are known.

Mantras can be easy, or they can be incredibly difficult—and if you're serious about healing through the use of mantras, you may want to consider contacting a qualified teacher that can help guide you to the most suitable mantra for you depending on where you are at in your journey and spiritual awakening. It is recommended that you start with a general mantra that can be used by anyone such as the "SO HUM" Mantra. Practice this by sitting comfortably with your eyes closed, and breathing normally. Begin repeating "SO" silently as you inhale, and repeat "HUM" as you exhale. Repeat this for 15-20 minutes. If you find your attention is drifting away or your thoughts are wandering, simply bring your attention back to the words. Practice saying the "HUM" out loud, and feel the energy of the sound as it escapes your body.

Mantras can be chanted aloud or repeated silently. They can create the desired effect in our life whether it's for healing, transformation, and/or inner awakening. Considered a "vedic science", mantras can take lifetimes to master. It's important to learn the correct pronunciation of each mantra, so if you are unsure of something, simply look it up! You don't have to be on a yoga mat or in a spiritual place to recite mantras. They are a tool that you can use anywhere and anytime that you might be feeling stressed, anxious, lonely, or excited. It's as easy as picking a word or phrase, even an invocation or affirmation that works for you. A rule of thumb is to repeat shorter mantras 108 times. Longer mantras may be repeated only a few times.

Let's explore some of the different types of and uses of mantras:

- **Om**

  The well-known sound that elicits visions of the Buddha or Hindu gods in the state of prayer, "Om" is known to be the first sound heard at the creation of the universe. Pronounced A-U-M, and when every syllable is fully pronounced, you should be able to feel the energy of the sound from your pelvic floor through the crown of your head. This droning sound is known for unblocking the throat chakra, and improves our communication with others.

- **Shanti/Peace Mantra**

  The short version is "Om santih, santih, santih". pronounced A-U-M, shanti, shanti, shanti, translated as "Om, Peace, Peace, Peace." This is performed literally, to increase the amount of peace in our lives. The longer version, which must be hard to pronounce properly, is translated to: "May there be well-being for all, peace for all, wholeness for all, and happiness for all."

- **Deity Mantra**

  Though there are thousands of deities in the Eastern traditions, those of us that are not so religiously inclined can view these deities as archetypal energies. All of these energies are within us, either in a balanced or imbalanced state. If they are dormant, we can experience a lack in that area, or a disruption, if they are unbalanced. When they are in harmony, we can enjoy fulfillment and harmony. A beginning deity mantra is "GAM" (gaam). This is used to remove obstacles and blockages, as well as for bringing wisdom into your life.

- **Healing Mantras**

Best learned from a qualified teacher, there are very powerful healing mantras. You are essentially reintroducing the correct sound to restore harmony. Repeated while focusing attention to the areas of discomfort, the goal is to direct the vibration to the areas the healing is needed. A few beginning healing mantras:

  o   Mmmmm—For the Sinus
  o   Nnnnnn—For the Ears
  o   Eeemmm—For the Eyes
  o   Gaa Gha—For the Throat
  o   Yaa Yu Yai—For the Jaw

You can also use the basic vowel sounds for healing, just direct the vibration where you want it to work (Aaa, Eeeee, Eye, Oooo, Uuu).

- **Chakra Mantras**

As we've learned, chakras are the energy vortexes within our bodies. Since mantras are directly working with our vibration, we can energize and align our chakras through their use. Below is a set of chakra meditations—be sure to go through all of them rather than just focusing on one or two. Start with the lowest, or first chakra, and work your way up. Repeat each sound a few times out loud or silently, and repeat daily.

- o LAAM—Root Chakra/associated with survival instincts
- o VAAM—Sacral Chakra/sensuality, creative inspiration
- o RAAM—Solar Plexus/ego, personal power
- o YAAM—Heart Chakra/compassion, unconditional love
- o KSHAAM—Third Eye Chakra/inspiration, insight
- o OMM—Crown Chakra/spiritual union

- **General Mantras**

To be used anytime we seek to enliven the qualities they bring forth with their vibration:

- o Santih (Shanti)—To restore harmony and peace

○ Anandam (Aan An Dam)—To restore contentment and inner joy

○ Om Bhur Bhuvah Suvaha (Om Bhoor Bhoo-va Su-va-ha)—For enlightenment

Again, this is just a glimpse into the extensive world of mantras as an Ayurvedic healing tool. Practice these, and experiment with mantras to see which ones you enjoy the most or receive the most benefit from. Memorize new ones as you continue on your journey to well-being.

Panchakarma

An Ayurvedic cleanse that restores body, mind, and spirit to a natural state of balance. This is an ancient practice and rejuvenation that is typically performed at a clinic or in a retreat setting. You can also experiment with panchakarma at home. Once you have determined your prominent dosha, you can tailor your experience to your individual needs. This should be done when you have a chance to escape the daily grind, and focus on your cleansing and healing. If you can rent a cabin in the woods, or somehow seclude yourself from your typical interactions, this will be much more effective. The goal is to spend most of your time in a state of relaxation, focusing on resting, walking in nature, and practicing gentle yoga and meditation. This process can release old, unresolved emotions that we store in our deep connective tissue. You may experience negative feelings and have the urge to suppress these emotions, but you should focus on resolving these emotions and working through them instead.

Day 1-3

Start by drinking 2 ounces of warm ghee in the early morning. Follow the diet that pacifies your dosha throughout the day. Finish the day with a triphala tea. This will act as a nourishing yet mild laxative. Follow this routine for the first three days.

Day 4-5

One these days of panchakarma, you will want to only eat kitchari for every meal. Drink a tea that is specific to your dominant dosha. For Vata, use equal parts ground ginger, cumin, and coriander. For Pitta, use equal parts cumin, coriander, and fennel. For Kapha, use equal parts ground ginger, cinnamon, and add a pinch of clove. At bedtime, during these 4 and 5 days, massage your body for at least 15-20 minutes with warm organic oil. Kapha—corn oil, Pitta—sunflower oil, and for Vata—sesame oil. Relax for a few minutes to allow your body to absorb the oil, and then take a hot bath or shower. Use natural soap to gently wash it off, but allow some oil to remain. Take a dose of triphala before heading to bed.

Day 6-8

Proceed with your regimen from days 4-5, but at bedtime, boil the herbal compound dashamoola (1 Tb to 2 Cups of Water). Once cooled, strain and use as a "basti", or an enema. Try your best to hold this in as long as you can, overnight if possible, but for at least 30 minutes.

Day 9-12+

Once you make it to day 9, you'll want to begin incorporating steamed vegetables to your kitchari. Gradually, you can begin to transition back to a heartier diet. Start by adding unyeasted bread and more vegetables. Over these 3-7 days, you'll want to adjust back to your doshic diet. Be sure to set aside time to rebuild your strength.

As you can see, you'll want to use this time as a purposeful period of rest. Practice Yoga and Meditation regularly for every day of the panchakarma. There are many retreats dedicated to this powerful Ayurvedic healing method. If you are able, you should seek out a retreat that aims to preserve and restore your health through these therapies. Traditionally, panchakarma is an almost month-long process to purify your body.

Chapter 4: Weight Loss through Ayurveda

We should use our capability for tasting like a tool to create harmony in our physical bodies and our emotional lives. To see food as medicine, we must use all sources of information, including signals from our tongue. It's important to pay attention to the biological signs and the psychological ones as well. Use your sense of taste as an emotional barometer. This is important for those of us that have attempted diet after diet without getting the results we want. If you're ready for a more holistic approach to weight-loss, Ayurveda can provide you with simple approaches that are easy to follow. On this journey, you'll be reclaiming your vibrant sense of health and well-being mentally, physically, and emotionally. It's important to understand that in Ayurveda, being overweight shows an inherent excess in the Kapha dosha. This may not be the only factor at play, but in Ayurveda, it's a huge piece of the puzzle. Think of the qualities of Kapha such as heavy, slow, cool, dense, soft, and substantive. Compare that to being overweight. A return to balance will require an increase of opposing influences including those that are hot, dry, rough, light, and sharp.

There are easy commitments that you can make to help achieve your ideal weight. While they may require discipline in the beginning, your body's natural intelligence will begin to surface and replace unhealthy cravings with more balanced urges. Work on these commitments until they become second nature.

Create a Routine

This can be the key to success using this Ayurvedic approach. By ensuring that these commitments become a natural part of our every day, we can develop supportive new habits. This sense of routine can soothe our nervous systems, reduce stress, and create a feeling of being more centered. You don't want to overcommit, so just start with the basics. Add on to your routine as you become familiar with the new rhythm.

- **Sleep Schedule**

  One of the best places to start when creating a daily routine for ourselves is by focusing on our sleep schedule. The Kapha time of day, or 6-10 p.m., is an ideal time to let our systems settle down and prepare to sleep. We want to align with the cycles of nature, and we can support this by finding an earlier bedtime—before 10 p.m. is ideal. Waking before the Kapha morning cycle between 6-10 a.m. is important as well. If we can wake up by 6 a.m., we can feel more alert and awake, since our body's metabolic capacity is supported. As we know, getting enough sleep is crucial to our health. We should consider our sleep and wake times together, so that we ensure that we are getting enough rest. You'll want to experiment with your sleep schedule to find the ideal number of hours you need to function at your optimal level. Adjust by 15 minutes at a time, and let a few days pass before making further changes. We must have consistency and discipline with our sleep and wake times so that we can truly move towards positive change.

- **Morning Yoga**

Set aside at least 15 minutes for yoga or physical stretching every day. If you do not make this a mandatory part of your day, it will most likely be forgotten. Schedule this around a part of your day when you can perform yoga on an empty stomach—typically early in the morning. This will elicit a relaxation response in your body, helping to alleviate stress. This can also help put us into a present state of mind where we can have better decision-making capabilities. Whether you always start by performing basic poses, or attempt those that are more challenging, the goal is to practice this meditative self-realization practice every morning.

- **Meal Time**

Eat your meals at the same time every day. Being consistent with mealtimes ensures enough space between meals, and reinforces that routine you need for a healthy metabolism and nervous system. Again, you'll want to experiment to find the ideal times for meals in your daily schedule. Aim to consume your lunch, which is typically the largest meal, between 11 and 2 p.m. when your digestive fires are the strongest. Focus on eating your dinner meal early and include light foods that are supportive of your weight-loss goals. In Ayurveda, eating only three meals a day is recommended. Intermittent fasting to rest your body and the digestive fire is also recommended. Listen to your body, and be sure to give it what it needs to function at its optimal levels. Every person is different, so you will be the best person to determine when you need to eat, and how much you need per day.

- **Exercise**

Schedule at least three days for exercise a week. Find ways that you can be active consistently throughout your days, especially those where you have no exercise scheduled. Having a predictable schedule can help you stick to your routine, and in turn, achieve your goals. Experiment with the best days and times for you to fit in physical exercise. Aim for at least 30-60 minutes of cardio activity, and if you are able, incorporate strength training into your workout routine. Your commitment to exercise should be in addition to your yoga practice. This commitment to exercise should be in addition to daily yoga practice. You'll want to look for physical activities that are fun for you, that invigorate you, and are doable. Even short workouts of only 15-20 minutes each time can be extremely beneficial, and easy to fit into the busiest of days. Plan your exercise around the times of day that will give you the best results. If you exercise during the Kapha times of day, the atmospheric conditions can help give a little extra strength and stamina to our systems. In Ayurveda, it's recommended that we exercise to 50-70% of our capacity. This means that we are ideally breathing through our nostrils the entire time. We want to prevent physiological stress, and allow our bodies to benefit more deeply from the effort.

A great method for getting the most out of your exercise time is high-intensity interval training (HIIT). This is a technique that alternates between short, intense bursts of activity and interspersed recovery periods. This allows our bodies to rest between these intense activity periods, and can be very useful when limited on time to dedicate for exercise. You simply warm up, and then perform a series of anywhere from 5-10 intervals of 30-60 second bursts of extreme activity, interspersed by recovery periods of 2-3 minutes. You can adjust the timeframes to fit where you are at physically. For example, on a treadmill, once you are warmed up, you can run as fast as you can for 30 seconds, and then reduce the speed to a slightly faster than normal rate until your next 30-second burst. This method has been shown to boost our metabolic function, reduce insulin resistance, burn fat, and support weight loss.

Even when you can't dedicate a lot of time, or even without a gym membership, you can find ways to be active at least 3 times a week. Start by walking or biking. Increase your intensity as your endurance increases. Listen to your body and pay attention to what it is telling you. While it's true that we must push past our comfort levels to see the results we desire, we must also remember to take care of our bodies and learn our own limitations. Create a workout routine around your needs, and commit to getting active.

- **Meditation**

Schedule quiet time for yourself. In Ayurveda, the power of subtle therapies is recommended. This could be paying attention to your emotional, psychological, and physical patterns that underly any imbalance in your life. It is known that emotional unrest is a factor in our eating habits and activity levels. Unprocessed emotions can interfere with our health and mental ability to care for ourselves. By creating a mindful practice, we can begin to neutralize the hold that patterns may have on our behaviors. If you're not a spiritual person or don't want to dedicate a lot of time to work on your inner self, simply aim for 10-15 minutes a day where you can practice "pranayama", also known as breathing exercises. This is a powerful way to access and reset longstanding patterns in our energetic bodies. There are many pranayamas that are suitable for weight-loss, but you may want to focus on those that clear stress, anxiety, and unresolved emotions such as "Nadi Shodhana", or alternate nostril breathing. There are many guided meditations and practices available online, which is great for beginners

Other tips for Ayurvedic Weight Loss

- Drink a large glass of warm water with lemon as soon as you wake up in the morning. This will boost your entire digestive system and give you a fresh start to the day.

- If you are able, find an activity that will cause you to break a sweat every morning. This will jump-start your fat-burning mechanism and give you energy.

- Eat with the seasons. Fresh fruits in the summer, and root vegetables and stored grains in the winter, our bodies naturally digest and assimilate nutrients when we eat foods that are found in the current season.

- Incorporate all six tastes. Take note of the foods you eat and their associated tastes. Use this to create a balance in your diet.
- Use the sun as a guide for bedtime. Start to wind down as the sun sets, aiming to get to bed before 10p.m. Rise with the sun and get a jump-start to your day.

Start with small steps. Ayurvedic healing will meet you where you are at now. The point is to create balance—not more stress in your life. If this is something you want to dive into headfirst, great, but it's okay to take small steps as well. Remember that we should find joy in eating and experiencing food. You should not allow a fear of gaining weight hold power over your joy of eating the food you love, as long as it's done in moderation. Ayurvedic healing regarding weight-loss doesn't need to involve any deprivation or hardship. Keep in mind the main law of Ayurveda—that like increases like. If you are getting heavier, it's likely that you have too many heavy qualities in your diet and lifestyle. This includes processed foods, meat, eggs, cheese, nuts, wheat, yogurt, milk, and alcohol. These foods are harder for the body to digest, and have heavy associations. These types of food contribute to our "ama", or undigested food wastes. When we have hampered digestion, our digestive fire can be dampened, as well as our tissue metabolism. This can turn into a negative cycle if we can't correct that digestive fire.

Consider gradual weight loss. This can be done by simply avoiding those heavy foods and increasing lighter foods. Provide your body with foods that are easy to digest and that keep the digestive fire burning. These foods include green vegetables, fruit as snacks, basmati rice, lentils, and spices such as coriander, ginger, and turmeric. Try starting with home-cooked vegetarian meals. Incorporate more soups for dinner, and try to make your heaviest meal at lunch. It's by making small adjustments that you get back into balance. Once you are back to your ideal balance, you can incorporate some heavy foods back in, if it is done in moderation. If you need to really kick start your weight-loss efforts, try to incorporate "moong daal", or mung beans into your main meals. This is recommended because mung beans are sweet and astringent, and are cooling too. They are light and dry, and balance the doshas while having a sattvic action on the mind. They are nourishing to the tissues and immune system, while also being light and easy to digest. Many feel that it fills them up while grounding them, but also leaves them feeling comfortable and well. A portion of great food for nourishing the body and the mind, mung bean is a staple in the Ayurvedic diet.

Another great recipe for weight loss is kitchari. Meaning "the mixture of two grains", kitchari is nourishing and easily digested.

There are many variations, but you can experiment to find the best combination for your tastes. "Mung dal", or split yellow beans, combined with Basmati rice, for example, create a balanced food that is tridoshic and has adequate amounts of protein. Kitchari is great for detoxifying and de-aging cells, and is elementary to the Ayurvedic way of being. Dating back thousands of years, kitchari incorporates spices and vegetables and makes a dish fitting for every lifestyle.

Ayurvedic Recipes

Whether your goal is to lose weight, maintain weight, or simply to improve your nutritional intake, following Ayurvedic recipes that align with your dominant dosha can be extremely beneficial for you. Let's review a few recipes that are tridoshic, or suited for all doshas. Remember the balancing of your daily meals should be remembered as "eat like a saint" for breakfast, "eat like a king" for lunch, and "eat like a pauper" for dinner.

Vegetable Curry (30 Minutes to 1-hour prep time)

- 1 Cup Green Peas
- 1 Cup Diced Carrots
- 1 Cup Diced Potatoes
- 2 Cups Asparagus or Green String Beans (Cut into Small Pieces)

- 2 Tb Oil (Ghee or Sunflower Oil)

- 2 Tb Mustard Seeds (Black)

- 1 teaspoon Salt (Himalayan Sea Salt or similar)

- 1 and ½ Cup Water (Purified)

- 2 tsp Turmeric

- 1 tsp Coriander

- ½ Cup Plain Yogurt (No Added Sweeteners)

Begin by heating the oil, and then adding in the cumin and mustard seeds. Add turmeric once those seeds start to pop, and then all of the vegetables and water. Covering the skillet, cook until vegetables are tender—typically 15 minutes. Add in the yogurt and remaining ingredients, taking care to incorporate all of them by stirring thoroughly. Simmer for an additional 15 minutes. This dish can be served over rice or other grains. Enjoy the cooling abilities of potatoes and peas in contrast to the spices.

Miso Tofu (15-20 Minutes prep time)

- 1 Lbs. Tofu

- 1 Tb Sunflower Oil

- ½ Onion-medium (Finely Sliced)

- 1 Tb Tamari

- ¾ Cup Water (Purified)

- 3 Mushrooms (Shitake)

- 1/8 teaspoon Black Pepper

Soak mushrooms in the water while warming oil in a skillet. Sauté onions until tender. Once the tofu is drained, cut into small cubes and add to the onion to sauté for 5 minutes. Sprinkle the black pepper over the tofu and onion. Drain the mushrooms, but save the water. Add the mushrooms to the skillet and mix in the tamari, water and the miso, and cover the tofu. Heat for an additional 5 minutes, then serve.

Rice and Dal

- ½ Cup Basmati Rice (Any Long Grain Rice Will Do)
- ¼ Cup Mung Dal (Mung Beans)
- 1 teaspoon Ghee
- ¼ tsp Cumin seeds
- 1/8 tsp Black Mustard Seeds
- 1 to 1 ½ Cups Water (Purified)

Place water, rice, and dal into a pot and boil. Separately, heat the ghee and mustard seeds until the seeds pop. Then, put in the cumin seeds and remove from the heat. Add this to the rice mixture and stir thoroughly. Reduce heat and simmer with a tight-fitting lid for 5-10 minutes before turning off the heat and allowing it to stand for another 30 minutes. Serve with steamed vegetables.

Porridge

The recipe for this breakfast porridge will vary depending on your personal taste and choice of ingredients. Traditionally, you will soak fruits such as dates, raisins, dried figs, and apricots in a pan of water overnight. Seeds such as sunflower, pumpkin, linseed, almonds, and shredded coconut can be added as well. When ready in the morning, you will boil this mixture and add to rolled oats or quinoa, barley flakes, or millet, cooling until soft. Add cinnamon powder and crushed cardamom seeds to taste. Add rice or almond milk to make a creamier version. If you need to sweeten it, add syrup such as a maple, or a fruit spread. This will provide the energy you need to make it through your morning and into your lunchtime meal.

In Ayurvedic eating, remember that the most important principle is that your food needs to be free from pesticides, additives, and other chemicals. It should be seasonal, and whenever possible, organic and local. This doesn't mean raw, however, as Ayurveda teaches that gently-cooked foods are more easily assimilated into our bodies. Experiment with these recipes, or research more to incorporate them into your diet. Making small adjustments like preparing food suited to your dosha is one of the best ways to begin your journey to well-being and health. Remember that eating should be enjoyable, and that you want to really take notice of every flavor, texture, and effect of everything you put into your body. Only then will you be able to determine which things you want to increase, and those you want to avoid.

Take a trip to your local farmers' market and see what foods are in season right now. Talk with a grower that sells herbs. Find online communities that share an interest in Ayurvedic knowledge and practice. There is a wealth of knowledge available on the subject, and many people are also just starting on their journey. Try ordering a triphala supplement, or attempt to make a tea to see what it is your taste. The next time you cook food using basil, try and find holy basil, or used dried tulsi to incorporate a bit of Ayurvedic medicine into your daily routine of making dinner. There is no right or wrong way to get started, but there is no better time than the present.

Conclusion

Congratulations for making it through till the end! Ayurvedic medicine and Ayurveda theory are extremely complex and diverse concepts, and should remain a part of your lifelong journey to optimal health and wellness. I hope this book provided you with the information you were seeking about how to apply some of the basic principles of Ayurveda into your daily life. The intent is for you to use this as a starting point, and a reference as you incorporate some of the techniques. From the surgical texts and compendium of the medical theory that came about in 800 BCE, to the growing popularity of Ayurvedic herbs in the Western World, Ayurveda is something that every generation becomes aware of to some extent. Remember, it's the study of life as a whole, and encompasses those basic instincts we all have for the attraction of pleasure and the repulsion for pain. Using this knowledge, you can start to apply lifestyle changes and develop a robust outlook for life.

It's important to consider the five elements and the ways that they encompass all our sensory organs. Everything that exists in the universe also exists within us as individuals. Those elements of the universe: Earth, air, fire, water, and ether/space manifest and exist in all of nature. Keep in mind that it's the three gunas that give rise to these elements. By understanding the gunas: Tamas, Rajas, and Sattva, we can understand our internal states and experiences. When there is an imbalance of these gunas, we experience disruptions in the normal functioning of our bodies. We should seek to promote Sattva qualities to clear the mind and restore balance. This is the foundation of Ayurvedic practice, that our body is inseparable from all other environments. As the gunas affect the creation and influence of the five elements, the five elements make up the three doshas, or bodily humor.

The three doshas are how each of us can assess our constitutions and the energetic forces behind our mind-body communication. To find our balanced states, we can take the appropriate action called for by our dominating dosha to eliminate those factors that keep us off balance. Vata, as the energies responsible for all movement, provides the essential motion for all our bodily processes. Pitta is known as that which cooks and shares many qualities of fire. Finally, Kapha, known as that which sticks, is the energies of lubrication and building. We must develop our awareness of our characteristics and traits to best determine the healing methods that will have the best effects for us. Look for other dosha tests online and compare all your answers when determining your dominant dosha. The Ayurvedic principle of the six tastes being used to form a balanced diet should be one of the first things you apply into your daily life. These tastes are therapeutic tools that have significant effects on our body, mind, and spiritual balance. There will be specific tastes that are better suited to your dosha, but you should experiment with all the tastes to create the best nutritional plan for yourself. Find something that you enjoy in every category: Sweet, salty, sour, pungent, bitter, and astringent.

Through rational, psychological, and spiritual therapies simultaneously, we can promote our healing process between our minds and bodies. Look at the practice of yoga as the physical extension of the Ayurvedic science of health. It is the combination of the two that can transform your existence by connecting you with the deep spiritual levels within yourself. This Ayurvedic self-healing and this yogic self-realization will help to understand the language of nature and life, and can lead to greater harmony between you and nature. Practice a few of the poses outlined in this book, seek others that match your dominant dosha as well, since it can be used to enhance Sattva. Promote health even further by acknowledging and balancing your chakras. By balancing your energetics, you will experience a higher awareness and harmony. Practice getting in touch with and understanding your chakras.

Explore other healing paths by experimenting with aromatherapy. Find aromas that you are drawn to, and that makes you feel well. A powerful Ayurvedic tool, aromatherapy and aromatic baths and massages can be especially beneficial when balancing your doshas. Try using some of the scents and oils recommended in this book for your dosha, and experiment with blending your favorite scents. Be sure to find ways to incorporate aromatherapy into your daily life,

even if it's just a diffuser on your work desk or incense at first.
Another powerful tool of Ayurvedic healing is herbal remedies.
Continue learning about the different herbs available in supplement
form, and those dried ones available for teas. Seek out those herbs
that you feel a connection with, or that you have an interest in, and
educate yourself to their healing properties. One of the best aspects
of Ayurveda is that almost anything can be used as a therapeutic tool.
Going further with this, every herb has a beneficial property. Test
out some of the common remedies mentioned, such as ashwagandha,
triphala, and curcumin. Experiment with herbs you can grow
yourself such as mint, basil, and thyme!

Use mantras to harmonize your natural vibrations, and experience a
feeling of wholeness. Start with a beginner mantra, and slowly
increase your dedicated time. As you continue your journey, seek out
mantras that fit into your place of spiritual awakening. Find mala
beads to help keep count, and dedicate yourself to practicing mantras
at least a few times a week. Meditative practices can have incredible
effects on our internal and external outlook, and a general sense of
wellbeing. Use the healing power of a panchakarma cleanses and
find balance by creating a nutritional plan for yourself that is focused
on balancing your dosha. Good luck to you on your journey, and
may you find the peace you seek.

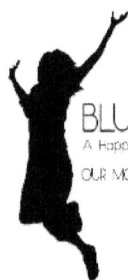

Connect with us on our Facebook page

www.facebook.com/bluesourceandfriends and stay tuned to our

latest book promotions and free giveaways.

Printed in Great Britain
by Amazon

32249087R00061